Accepting Life

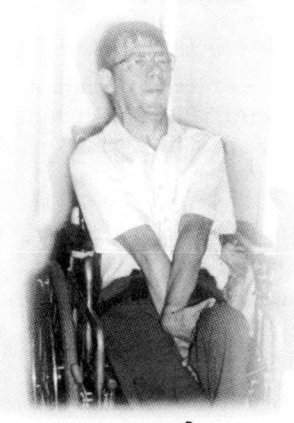

acceptinglife

GERRY PETERSON

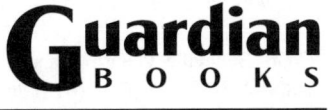

Belleville, Ontario, Canada

ACCEPTING LIFE
Copyright © 2005, Gerry Peterson

All Rights Reserved. No part of this publication may be reproduced, stored in a retrieval system or transmitted in any form or by any means—electronic, mechanical, photocopy, recording or any other—except for brief quotations in printed reviews, without the prior permission of the author.

All Scripture quotations, unless otherwise specified, are taken from the HOLY BIBLE, NEW INTERNATIONAL VERSION ®. Copyright © 1973, 1978, 1984 by International Bible Society. Used by permission of Zondervan Publishing House. All rights reserved. • Scripture quotations marked NKJV are taken from the New King James Version. Copyright © 1979, 1980, 1982. Thomas Nelson Inc., Publishers. • Scripture quotations marked KJV are from *The Holy Bible, King James Version.* Copyright © 1977, 1984, Thomas Nelson Inc., Publishers.

Library and Archives Canada Cataloguing in Publication

Peterson, Gerald F. (Gerald Fredrick), 1949-
  Accepting life / Gerald F. Peterson. -- 2nd ed.

First ed. published Edmonton : Coldham Press, 1988 under title:
  Accepting reality.
ISBN 1-55306-924-2

  1. Peterson, Gerald F. (Gerald Fredrick), 1949- 2. Cerebral palsied--Canada--Biography. 3. Christian biography--Canada.
I. Peterson, Gerald F. (Gerald Fredrick), 1949- . Accepting reality.
II. Title.

RC388.P48 2005   362.196'836'0092   C2005-902580-8

For more information or
to order additional copies, please contact:
Gerald F. Peterson
CHRIST-ABLED (Gerry's Ministry)
14407 McQueen Rd.
Edmonton, Alberta T5N 3L3 Canada
E-mail: gerrypet@telusplanet.net

Guardian Books is an imprint of *Essence Publishing,* a Christian Book Publisher dedicated to furthering the work of Christ through the written word.. For more information, contact:

20 Hanna Court, Belleville, Ontario, Canada K8P 5J2.
Phone: 1-800-238-6376 • Fax: (613) 962-3055
E-mail: publishing@essencegroup.com
Internet: www.essencegroup.com

Table of Contents

Preface 7

CHAPTER 1   Maternal Instinct 9
CHAPTER 2   My Working Tools 17
CHAPTER 3   The Group Home Battle 27
CHAPTER 4   Growing Up Spiritually 33
CHAPTER 5   Accepting My Relationships 39
CHAPTER 6   All Things Work Together for Good ... 49
CHAPTER 7   Trials & Testings 53
CHAPTER 8   Attitudes 63
CHAPTER 9   At Heaven's Gate 67
CHAPTER 10 Accepting Reality 71

Preface

This book is an update of my first book, which was written about twenty-five years ago about my life. A great deal has happened during my life journey, including some very special relationships. The story reveals struggles, pain, and misunderstandings caused by other people who do not know all the facts. Since I am writing this from a Christian perspective, I want to encourage others to know that God is working out His plan even when it may appear that the world has fallen apart.

I would like to thank God, my King and Saviour Jesus Christ, that I have been given this life, which I have been able to live in the midst of storms and circumstances that are not easily understood.

I am thankful also for my parents, my two brothers, my nephew and two nieces and their spouses and children, for including me as the recipient of their love and care. My father taught me so much about life. My mother was the one who demonstrated her faith in me and took upon herself the task of fighting for the rights and needs of the disabled community. Mom taught me to be an independent person.

I also want to thank my family for their personal faith in God and their willingness to make sure that I attended church, where I was able to hear the gospel and learn about the forgiveness and love of God. They allowed me to make my own choices in life, as I progressed on my journey to becoming a man.

I want to express my thanks to my friend Dick Paetzel for his wisdom and help in the development of this book. I also want to thank Anne and Wes Kruger for reviewing the manuscript, obtaining a readable form.

I want to dedicate this book in loving memory to my sweetheart and friend Tammy Lee Miller.

GERALD F. PETERSON

One

Maternal Instinct

My name is Gerry Peterson, and I would like to tell you, my reader, the story of my life. This book is written as a window into my life, from the perspective of overcoming cerebral palsy, beginning with my very first gasp for air.

The hours that preceded my arrival into this world, on a cold but sunny Sunday, were indeed anxious ones. My mother instinctively knew something was wrong as she drifted in and out of semi-consciousness. Some hours later she learned I had been without oxygen for twenty minutes. A nun in charge of the delivery room had alerted the off-duty nurses to pray in the chapel—to pray for baby Peterson and his mom's life. Mother Superior came to visit my mother and, even though they had differing views on matters of theology, the nuns could not shirk their responsibilities. I was not expected to live, so they baptized me and committed me to the Lord. So you see, I was ushered into this world on "the wings of prayer."

Mom hovered between life and death for three days, but when, at last, she was able to hold me and touch my tiny

Accepting Life

hands for the first time, Mom's heart was overflowing with thanks that they, my parents, had their first son—in the person of Gerald Frederick Peterson.

As new parents, they spent weeks and months of disturbed nights, due to my being ill a great deal. Upon reflection, her professional training as a nurse should have alerted Mom to the signals that were being sent out, but her mothering instinct somehow refused to pick up on those signals.

When I was seven and a half months old, Mom took me to a pediatrician for a check-up. He carefully examined me and afterwards told her to dress her son. The doctor sat behind a large desk and kept twirling a pair of glasses around. Sensing his inability to find the place to start, Mom finally picked up the courage to say, "Okay now, tell me what is wrong with my baby."

He sat silently for what seemed an eternity and then replied, "He has Little's disease (cerebral palsy). He will be hopelessly crippled. My advice to you is that you put him in an institution and forget that you ever had him."

The room was oppressively still. She grabbed me with my blanket and jumped up screaming. "Oh no, I won't! Over my dead body, neither you nor anyone will put this child in an institution."

Mom doesn't remember how we got home, but somehow she had found a bus. When we arrived, my dad was already home from work. Through her distress, she managed to tell my dad the diagnosis, and they both wept.

It wasn't until a little later that the shock set in. Mom shed many tears for me, arguing and bargaining with God, wrestling with non-acceptance of the fact that I indeed did have cerebral palsy. Oh yes, my mother at times berated God's apparent injustice. "Why you, our beautiful son with blue eyes...no, it couldn't be." She felt sorrow such as she had never known before; she grieved that her son should be so afflicted.

But, praise God, my dad dealt with his grief in a different way and was Mom's rock and support. Their love for me knew no bounds. My smile and eyes captivated them all. My parents prayed that God would prove the doctor to be wrong—that somehow they would wake up one morning and find it was all a bad dream. It was all to no avail. Mom did a lot of soul searching during these times. She was ridden with guilt. When she held me, and she held me a lot because of my fretting, she would ask herself, "What terrible sin have I committed that contributed to this tragedy?" Through all of this they loved me dearly.

Mom prayed; she cried; she screamed and lashed out at God; but she searched the Scriptures for guidance and answers...but answers to what? Where could Mom go for the solace she was so desperately seeking?

They prayed that God would change things, knowing all the while they must accept what had happened to their baby. Through it all they continued loving me. I grew month by month. My eyes would tell them when I was happy or when I was sick. It is often said that eyes are the windows of the soul, and my parents learned a lot about me during those times. From what they saw in those eyes, no one would convince them that their boy was not capable of understanding or learning.

Mom wrote everywhere for information on cerebral palsy and, in those days (almost fifty years ago), there was precious little to be found. The Minister of Health for the Province of Alberta denied there were any children with cerebral palsy in Alberta. Mom wrote back and announced

Accepting Life

that we now had one and asked what was going to be done about it! The "official" ignorance and stupidity regarding this affliction was incredible.

I was susceptible to respiratory ailments and had pneumonia several times before my first birthday. Little by little, mother and baby formed their routine of eating, sleeping, playing, growing and living. But inside my mom the battle always raged! "Why, God? Why this child, why this mother?" Over and over she asked those questions: day and night—night and day. Cerebral palsy! It coloured their days and disrupted their nights. The tiny muscle spasms, the lack of coordination—to the extent that I could not hold a rattle, a bottle or a spoon—caused total frustration for all of us as the storms of unanswered questions raged on. "Why, God, why?" But my parents were not alone; as the grandparents, aunts and uncles each heard that this newest, much loved member of the family had cerebral palsy, there was disbelief and, in most cases, abysmal ignorance. Each reacted in his own way. My grandfather and grandmother Bohlman were grief stricken and did all they could to offer comfort over the years. They loved me in a very special way, always supporting and always praying that God would hold me in His hand.

My mom and dad were proud of me and took me everywhere, often to my consternation. At that time, society basically ignored the disabled, regardless of their disability. There were no government programs, no special schools, in fact, no real support—even the church was at a loss in these matters. Nevertheless, when I was nine months old, my parents dedicated me, as well as themselves, to God before the congregation of His people.

During those early months—amid all the turmoil, the tears, the searching for answers to questions Mom could hardly articulate—God granted a serenity that broke through like a rainbow after a storm. She knew life for her would never be the same. Society would have to be forced to change. People would have to be made aware of the realities of birth injuries. Somehow, and she did not know how, she would have to play a part in breaking down those barriers. The old prejudices and ignorance had to go! She had no idea of how difficult, or how long, this assignment would be, but between God, Gerry and herself, they were going to change a lot of things.

As time passed, my two younger brothers arrived to be part of our family, and one of the expressions they learned at an early age was "cerebral palsy." I joined in all their games and played with all the neighbourhood children. Afterwards they would ask mom, "Why can't Gerry walk?" or "Why can't Gerry talk?" The answer that stopped them cold was "cerebral palsy." Children accept children and make allowances for disabilities, which sometimes adults would do well to copy.

When I was about ten years old, my dad had a walker made for me, so I could play with my two brothers and our friends on the street. They, too, wanted to know why I could not walk and talk, so they asked my mom or their mothers, "Why can't Gerry walk?"

My parents pushed me to be independent. Often I decided to go around our block by myself in my walker. Many times the neighbour ladies called my mom to tell her where I was, or would push me home, because I was just a disabled child. When they phoned my mom, she replied, "Do you know where your children are?" I'm sure those ladies thought my mother was crazy for letting her disabled boy go around the block by himself with a walker.

One special relationship was with my dog, whom my father found at the city dog pound. Jet, as I affectionately knew him, was two years old then. The first time I tried to pet him, my hand closed up with his hair in my hand and, try as I might, I couldn't release my grip! So I ended up pulling out his hair. He responded by biting my arm, because he didn't understand. The next time I pulled his hair, he just yipped, then gave me a kiss! If someone came too near to me, he would let them know it was time to back away.

Once I asked Dad to tie my dog to my walker. For the first few minutes, Jet pulled me slowly. But then he saw a cat! The road was under repair, so there was a metre drop-off, which the cat had no problem crossing. Jet and I did not do as well. A tangled mess of steel, fur and boy explained the need to hurry to the hospital. When my parents returned from the hospital, on the front steps were a sad company of neighbourhood kids, my two little brothers and especially a dog needing to be consoled. When I got back from the hospital, I went to Jet to let him know that I was okay. He was happy to see me again, and my dad told me that he wouldn't tie Jet to my walker again.

My dog often went away for a few nights before deciding it was time to come back home. The city pound called so many times for my parents to come and get him, I am sure they knew our phone number by heart!

On one such occasion, Jet had been away for five days. My parents concluded something terrible must have happened to him. On the fifth night, however, I heard him, but

Maternal Instinct

when I told my parents, they didn't believe me. The next morning when we were coming back from church, Dad started to tell us he thought the dog was probably dead, but Mom suddenly saw Jet running. So Dad stopped the car and called him; the dog bounded in on top of us, bringing with him a ton of dirt! It was then they realized I had actually heard my dog the night before. Needless to say, the dog needed washing!

My mother's battle with God raged on over a period of about ten years. The bargaining continued: "God, if only he could walk by the time he is five years old...if only he could talk by age six." God must have smiled at all these "if onlys"; after all, who was she to bargain with the great and sovereign God? Mom was just a desperate mother who loved her son more than life itself. However God, through His Word, gradually revealed His truth to her, and she learned that His love and grace were sufficient.

And then one day she finally accepted the fact that cerebral palsy was here to stay in their lives. It was a sunny fall day. She had left the three boys with their father and gone downtown to shop. She can still see how the sun shone through the bus windows, as she made her way home laden with packages. Suddenly she was filled with an indescribable feeling of peace, and she remembers praying "God, I can now accept what has happened to Gerry. I commit all this to you. Now give me the strength to go on from here."

The bus made its routine stops; people boarded very much pre-occupied with their own problems. Mom felt very detached from all that was going on around her, yet was elated that she at long last had taken her burden of anger, frustration, guilt, denial and bargaining to Him. She accepted the fact that, just as He promised in His Word, He would uphold her. Mom had no idea what lay in store for the family, but with the burdens finally laid to rest, she knew life, both hers and mine, could be lived to the fullest.

Two

My Working Tools

When I was eleven years old, Mom and I were going through a difficult time trying to come up with a simpler method of communication. We had relied on the twenty-question method, the animal and vegetable kingdoms, the process of elimination, communication by gestures, guessing and even just gut feelings; but there had to be a better way. My parents knew I could read at a level appropriate to my age. We had gone over my vocabulary, and I was learning new words with a good comprehension level. But it was still difficult to communicate with my friends, family, teachers and classmates.

This trial and error process continued over a period of several years; Mom had tried every imaginable concept. Nothing was satisfactory, and I was still unable to express my deepest needs and desires. The combined frustration level was off the charts. No solution to this terrible dilemma was even remotely in sight. Each new idea had to be discarded for one reason or another. Mom prayed constantly for some insight, some clue, some workable solution. She knew there was an answer, but would we find it?

Accepting Life

We must be missing the obvious. She cried aloud to God. "God, I've had it; I can't help Gerry in this crucial area. I'm angry, disheartened and thoroughly exhausted by this whole problem, so God you'd better show me what I am to do, because I have run out of ideas. We are tired, and it's over and out, so you take over Lord." Mom wept as she went about her daily tasks. Her strength was completely spent. Two days went by, and she waited for the Lord to open her eyes to what she felt must be obvious. Once again after supper dishes were done, Mom lifted her sorrowing heart to the Lord and thanked Him for listening to her, for understanding her anxious spirit and for upholding her with His right hand. She sat down in the living room and began reading the evening paper.

Suddenly, the atmosphere of the evening changed as she saw it! Mom jumped up, yelling, "I've got it! I've got it! I've got the answer; Oh thank you Lord! Oh thank you Lord!" My brothers came running. She excitedly explained what God had shown her. As Mom had sat reading the newspaper, she "saw" individual words. She realized that we could take the often-used words of my vocabulary and list them alphabetically. Then, by pointing to words, I could communicate. Mom and I devised and revised many word sheets, but at least now I could choose my own words and communicating was beginning to be truly mine.

When I was thirteen, our family moved to Saskatoon. My father was an officer in the RCMP. It was a sad and disruptive time for me, for there were many changes in my life. Saskatoon, however, seemed friendlier almost immediately because of the purchase of a brown puppy that my brother and I found in a pet shop and promptly pressured our parents into buying.

Before we had moved, Dad told us that we could not have any pets in a rental house in Saskatoon, because the RCMP wouldn't allow it. So Dad found a farm that offered to take Jet and give him a good home. This allowed Jet to run free.

But when we saw our new home for the first time, my brothers and I saw two dogs and fish tanks. One of my brothers asked the renter if the RCMP allowed pets in this house, and he answered yes. The next day, Brian, my youngest brother, pushed me in my wheelchair to a mall, where we found a pet shop with many puppies. We especially liked one little puppy who licked my hand; Brian and I asked our parents to come look at the puppy. Our family was staying in a hotel until the other family moved out. Probably, my parents thought they couldn't buy a puppy when we were staying in a hotel, but the owner told Dad he was willing to hold the puppy until we moved into our new home. Dad asked us if we were willing to take care of this dog. We naturally agreed to look after this puppy, so Dad bought the newest member of our family with a smile on his face. When we went back to the hotel, Mom asked us what we should name the puppy. My brothers threw many names out to Mom; after a few minutes Mom said let's call her Taffy, because of her colour, and we agreed. Taffy became my constant companion and confidant for thirteen years.

May I add this footnote: I still miss my dogs. Jet was the better of the two dogs I had. They both gave me great pleasure as they learned to obey my commands. I especially enjoyed telling them to run away, just to see them express a freedom that was not mine. My parents could never understand why my dogs always ran away!

Accepting Life

Saskatoon had an excellent school for disabled children. Shortly after our arrival Mom and I went for an interview. That school was to change my life in a most profound way.

I was excited but could not believe my eyes when we pulled up in front of this dear old World War II hanger. It was originally built for housing planes and equipment but was to be my new school. It had been converted to a suitable space and housed an elevator that could well have served Noah's Ark. It was that large and moved just as slowly.

My fears disappeared as I found Dr. B. was a very special person, who immediately put me at ease. I felt as if I had known him all my life after being in his presence for only a short time.

I remember his telling me that I would be able to use a typewriter by Christmas. Frankly, I thought he was joking, and the disbelief must have shown in my eyes. One of my schoolmates said, "If Dr. B. said it, then it will be!" To my total surprise and satisfaction, two weeks before Christmas I was using a typewriter and was actually beginning to believe the doctor.

For Christmas my parents gave me an old IBM typewriter; it was then the real struggle began! I nearly swept it away with the river of my tears. Eventually I did learn to type, with a wand attached to a headband, which gave birth to my word board. My mother, who was instrumental in the original design, tells the following story:

> This all was pretty heady stuff for both of us; not all of the frustration was overcome, nor all the tears dried up; however, we knew we were on the right track. We struggled with this cumbersome equipment for a couple of years until once again God moved on our behalf.

My Working Tools

The teachers all felt Gerry could learn to type, but how? He tried to hold a stick between his teeth, but that was too awkward. The best-controlled muscles were in the neck, but how could we best utilize them? Everyone worked at finding a solution. Various things were tried and yet rejected as unsuitable.

By then, Gerry was thirteen years old, and an answer to this problem was crucial to his progress in school. It was a warm fall afternoon. On our front lawn was a city work crew digging up the nice green grass, for some reason best known to them. I was busy at the kitchen sink talking to God about my particular need. I had just finished giving Him an epistle on how I had exhausted my resources, telling Him the teachers had no answer to this dilemma either.

Glancing out of the window, I noticed one of the workmen had removed his hard hat and was holding it in such a way that the inside was visible. "Oh! There is my answer!" I raced outdoors to the workman and said, "Please, may I see your hat?" He looked bewildered but handed it to me. I took it and ran to the house, calling back, "I'll bring it right back; I need to make a phone call." By now, all the digging on the lawn came to a screeching halt.

I phoned the school and asked for Dr. B. When he came to the phone, all I could say was "I found it...I found it."

"Found what?" he asked.

"I found the answer of how to attach the wand to a headpiece."

That plastic band inside the hard hat became the key to our success. Mom's idea was that if we could attach a wand

Accepting Life

to the headpiece and devise a strap for under the chin, I would be able to type. We were overjoyed. Mom returned the hard hat and explained the magnificent discovery. All they could say was "Well I'll be...!"

A short time later the headpiece was a reality. It was made and worn like a hat, with a chinstrap to hold it in place and a wand firmly attached to the front. I took it to the typewriter, and a complete new world of communication opened up for me. Oh, how we thanked God for His goodness.

My dad and I then devised a portable word board. Using two pieces of plywood and a piano hinge, we made the board to fit my wheelchair; on the board were some 200 words and phrases as well as a "typewriter" keyboard alphabet. Now I could really communicate with the world around me, by pointing to the words or spelling them out on the keyboard.

The word board, headpiece and typewriter became my tools. None of it came easily, but I learned to make my "stubborn" body co-operate with these new devices. The struggles were hard, the tears many, but the rewards were tremendous, since I now had independence in thought and word.

A few years later Dr. B. told some of us that one day we would have a box that would be able to speak for us. What he described to us was small enough to carry on our wheelchairs. The staff thought he was crazy, but we believed in Dr. B., because each time he said something, somehow it came into being. I remember the first machine, which could type one word using only two keys. It was as large as a couple of refrigerators with a typewriter attached. I remember one very important thing Dr. B. told me: never use the word *can't*. Today I believe I would have learned to walk if I had been born in Saskatoon and stayed under his care. And he

My Working Tools

was right: today I have a computer, which gives me so much more freedom and independence.

At camp one summer, when I was sixteen or seventeen, I heard that Dr. B. had died. It didn't hit me until September when I went back to school. I was hoping that in some way it was just a bad dream. I was upset with God and really did not give the new doctor a chance. I really felt lost without Dr. B. Early one morning, just before we moved back to Edmonton, I thought I saw Dr. B. standing by the foot of my bed. I distinctly recall his words to me that everything would be fine. Despite what I was taught in Sunday school, that ghosts came from the Devil, I know whom I saw in my bedroom that morning.

My youngest brother had a weekly paper route. One spring day, Brian told me that I could not have a paper route, because I was in a wheelchair. I thought I would show him that a disabled person in a wheelchair could most certainly have a weekly paper route. So, I made a sign-up sheet on my typewriter; it said "Starting in September I will have a weekly paper route on Tuesday in the school clinic. Whoever is interested to get that weekly from me, please sign up." About twelve staff signed up, and in September a few more persons decided to take that paper from me. I delivered the paper in a nice warm building, while my brother and the other children had to deliver in all kinds of weather. I delivered the *Monday Paper* on Tuesdays for two years! Now he never says I can't do something!

Our family started camping in 1954, a holiday that in those days was for rich Americans and foolish people. Our neighbours thought my parents were half crazy to take their two older sons camping; they left Brian with our grandparents for three weeks, because he was just two. In the 1950s Banff and Jasper were very wild; we could see many bears, deer, elk and other wild animals. I enjoyed seeing them run wild and free. Now Banff and Jasper are not only for nature lovers but cater to the almighty dollar; I am sorry for that.

We first had a small tent, then a larger tent, then my father made a tent trailer, which we enjoyed for around six years. Then we bought a small trailer and then a larger trailer, for a few summers. This took place over twenty summers—summers that I really enjoyed.

I remember an experience when I was around six years old; we were camping by a lake at Jasper. We had been at a National Park movie, because it was dark when my dad lifted me over his head, and I saw a beautiful picture around me. It was the last few moments of daylight, because I saw the sunlight on a tip of a mountain next to a black night sky with a billion silver stars and the dark forest with its wonderful sounds around me. I was full of amazement when I looked on God's creation. It was very peaceful because I knew that I was safe in my father's hands, so I could enjoy that moment with him.

I felt as David did when he wrote in one of his psalms:

The heavens declare the glory of God; the skies proclaim the work of his hands. Day after day they pour forth speech; night after night they display knowledge. There is no speech or language where their voice is not heard. Their voice goes out into all the earth, their words to the ends of the world. In the heavens he has pitched a tent for the sun, which is like a bridegroom coming forth from his pavilion, like a champion rejoicing to run his course. It rises at one end of the heavens and makes its

My Working Tools

circuit to the other; nothing is hidden from its heat (Psalm 19:1–6).

Every time we left the mountains I cried, and my two younger brothers loved to make fun of me. I realized that I would miss all of this nature, which I had enjoyed and still enjoy today.

When I was fifteen, I asked Brian, my youngest brother, to turn the TV off because the station was off the air. Saskatoon had only one station then, and I wanted to save some electricity. But, Brian did not turn the TV off, so I was mad at him because he didn't obey me. I stood up from my wheelchair, and my brother was amazed I could stand up. But I remembered that I could not stand up; I fell to the floor and injured my left arm. It was just a few days before our holiday. My parents took me to the hospital to see if I had broken my arm, which I had. So I had a cast on when we went on our holidays.

My brother Brian and I, with two younger friends, went on an old logging trail that was going up the mountain. Going up was okay, but when we wanted to go back down the mountain, my chair kept going faster and faster, and I was unable to control it. I flew out of my chair and landed on some moss. I opened my eyes, looked up and saw my wheelchair fly above me.

Dad noticed some blood in my hair, so he asked me what happened on the mountain. I told him nothing had happened on the mountain. Then, Dad went to Brian, asked him the same question and Brian gave the same answer. Then, Dad went to the girl of the group, asked her the same question, and she gave the same answer. Finally, he went to the youngest member of the group, who was just four years old. He played with him and the boy's dead fish in a Dairy Queen dish. Dad asked him what happened on the mountain; the boy told him that he should have seen Gerry flying, because it was funny.

Three

The Group Home Battle

As I grew older my parents encouraged me to be independent in spite of my physical limitations. It seems that in this they succeeded beyond their wildest expectations.

Already at nineteen, I wanted to "get out of the nest." My parents were increasingly aware that as I came to the end of my teen years, the day would come when, because of their age and infirmity, they would be unable to care for my physical needs.

The option for a lifestyle in which I could truly exercise my personal freedoms was non-existent. Society's only option for physically disabled young adults was placing them in nursing homes for the elderly. It was our strong conviction this was no solution to an ever-growing problem. More and more disabled children were growing to adulthood through better medical care and research. Society was offering nothing new by way of suitable living accommodations.

By the end of the '60s, several group homes for physically disabled but mentally alert young adults began to be built in England. Mom began meeting with people who saw the necessity of such homes in Canada. In Saskatoon, where we were living at the time, a group formed to attempt a pilot project. Planning began in spite of severe opposition from the government, whose only solution to the problem was to institutionalize everyone that required special living accommodations and care.

It was our sincere conviction that what I needed was a home, in every sense of the word, where I, and those like me, could have our own personal space, with one bedroom for each resident. It should be a residence built on a non-medical model. It should have full-time staff to assist with personal care for each individual, with cooking and various household tasks that could include the involvement of the residents. We also undertook to prove this could be done with less funding than was required in an institutional setting.

The battle lines were drawn. There were meetings and more meetings, until eventually some progress was made. Capital costs were to be realized by private funding, whilst maintenance costs would be covered by the government. There was only one snag. It had never been attempted in Canada, and, unfortunately, the wheels of the government grind exceedingly slowly, and bureaucracy is firmly entrenched in the status quo, all of which generated more meetings. However, we all remained quite hopeful.

Our first glimmer of hope came from the Alberta Rehabilitation Council for the Disabled (ARCD). One staff member was very sympathetic to our cause and allowed Mom to present our dream to anyone in the organization that would give us a hearing. Later Mom was appointed to the ARCD Board of Directors (later to be named "The March of Dimes"). This position enabled her to present many recommendations as well as educate various community groups, Social Services and government agencies. It was a struggle of enormous proportions to gain support for these living accommodations. The opposition took many approaches: "Was it really necessary?" "Was it feasible?" "How, and by whom, would such a home be funded?" "Could it really be done?" On and on went the questions, each one having to be addressed, since we had no models to follow.

The break through came in 1970 when the ARCD was the beneficiary of the Milton Elmer Elves Estate, and in 1972 we made a submission to the executor regarding the building of a group home in Edmonton. The submission was accepted, and the group home was to be a pilot project.

A Planning Advisory Committee was formed, which comprised of members from the community with expertise in many areas. That began a series of events where each step had to be assessed, which brought about many changes in the plans. In all this, it was necessary to gain community and government support. Most watched with much skepticism. The staff at the ARCD was our main line of encouragement, support and guidance. Scores of ideas were looked at, accepted and rejected; many meetings attended, and many battles won and lost.

Eventually Mom accepted the position of coordinator for the group home project, which meant she became even more involved. This resulted in a toll on her health and a badly needed knee surgery. She would have discontinued her involvement had it not been for a dear friend who argued too much time and labour had been expended by her just to turn the project over to someone else.

After a long and arduous process that involved the city of Edmonton, the Minister of Social Services, his staff and a supportive community, it was agreed to build the group home on McQueen Road. In the late fall of 1974, Mom had the privilege of turning the sod at the site.

Many were the arguments put forth to our committee regarding the necessity of making this a home for six persons. The government wanted twelve, thus we compromised and settled for a nine bedroom home, each resident having a private room. In retrospect, it is both amusing and disturbing to note the latest government trends in building and funding group homes for the mentally disabled have been tailored for four to six occupants!

My mom knew that by giving young, physically disabled persons the opportunity to prove they could live in an independent environment, we were setting a precedent for those who were to follow. Since that time, many group homes have been built in Canada and many other types of living accommodations have been established.

Now thirty years later, many residents, past and present, have found the group home to be a stepping stone to further independence. Those who have made it their home have proved beyond a doubt that with proper and adequate support services, the concept we established was both right and justified. We are happy and proud that the group home has allowed me a real sense of personal freedom.

Now looking back, there were times when Mom felt completely overwhelmed by the project and the process, but somehow God supplied the strength when it was most needed. There are always those within society who are afraid to be creative and innovative. They will always be among us; they disagree and are disagreeable, because they do not understand those of us who dream of better ways to do those tasks that need to be done. I thank God she had the privilege of being a part of establishing a home that offered more than any institution. It was a dream come true.

One special verse of Scripture, which helped sustain us throughout that whole era, is found in Proverbs 31:8,9: *"Speak up for those who cannot speak for themselves, for the rights of all who are destitute. Speak up and, judge fairly; defend the rights of the poor and needy."*

Four

Growing Up Spiritually

I know that I am a child of God. I know Jesus Christ as my Lord and Saviour. My earliest recollections are those of my parents teaching me about God and His Son, Jesus Christ. All through my formative years, I was nurtured by Christian parents and Sunday school teachers. In our home God is honoured and worshiped. The Scriptures are regarded as truth and Jesus acknowledged as the Son of God. As to the exact time I asked Him to be my personal Saviour and friend, I cannot really say.

I used to think a holy God would not accept me because of my physical body. I do not know where I got that idea, but I do remember an early Sunday school teacher who had a crippled hand. She taught me that God does not look at our physical bodies but at our hearts. Some time later, I started to wonder how I could ask Jesus to come into my life and be my Lord and Saviour—I would guess that I was eight or maybe nine years old at the time.

For the next few years I was thinking whether or not I should give my life to God or not. My moods were up and down, hot and cold, believing and doubting. I do not know when the Lord actually became a real part of my life, because there was no Damascus Road experience, no bells, no angelic voices, just the constant assurance that the acceptance of Christ's love and forgiveness was the most important decision I would be expected to make. I recognized my great need for a personal Saviour and that I was a sinner in need of God's forgiveness. Eventually I did accept Jesus into my life to be Lord and director in everything.

I learned at and early age the Bible truth that *"God so loved the world that He gave His only begotten Son, that whoever believes in Him should not perish, but have everlasting life"* (John 3:16 NKJV). It followed that I could accept Him, who said, *"I am the way, the truth and the life. No one comes to the Father except through me"* (John 14:6 NKJV).

As a family we often attended church summer camps; these afforded us many happy hours of shared experiences with our friends. At one particular camping season, I was really moved by the Holy Sprit to explore the meaning of, and to seek, baptism. At first, I dismissed the strong urging as "emotionalism" due to the setting, but the feeling persisted and grew stronger.

One minister must have sensed my deep longing, for he discussed first with my parents and then with me the possibility of my being baptized. I expressed my desires to my family and pastor. Mom spent time discussing baptism, its meaning and significance, so that we could assess my understanding of the step I was about to take.

As was customary in our church, two deacons came to our home to conduct an interview as to the suitability of my candidacy. I was able to convey to them my beliefs and that I understood *"Or don't you know that all of us who were baptized into Christ Jesus were baptized into his death? We were therefore buried with him through baptism into death in order that, just as Christ was raised from the dead through the glory of the Father, we too may live a new life"* (Romans 6:3,4).

When I was eighteen, I was approached by my doctor to consider a surgical procedure known as trepanning. A rotating disc would be put into the skull, and pressure within the skull would be relieved, in the hope that this would lessen the uncontrollable movements of my arms and legs.

The doctor and I discussed the procedure at some length; the pros and cons were reviewed. The incidence of success was questionable, and there was the danger of becoming more limited on one side of my body. Many family discussions were held, but in the final analysis, I was left to make the ultimate decision. What dreadful days those were. One day I was convinced and wanted it done, but the next moment I wavered and would decide "no."

Finally a final decision had to be made. I consented and was placed on the waiting list for a hospital bed for this elective surgery. I thought how great it would be to have more control over my spastic limbs, and so I waited. Daily I agonized, drawing my whole family into my deliberations.

Several weeks passed and, at a time I least expected it, the hospital called. It was a beautiful sunny Easter morning; the snow was almost gone in Saskatoon. Dad and I had stayed at home that Sunday and I was on my bed listening to the radio when Dad came into my room and said, "Are you ready to go to the hospital, son?" Panic struck, what was I to do? "O God help me" was my earnest plea.

My schoolmates were somehow looking to me to provide answers for them in the event they might also consider

Accepting Life

this surgery. The procedure had not been done for a cerebral palsy victim in that city. Feelings of anxiety and hope competed for my attention.

Mom and my two brothers returned from church. Once again I began to have misgivings and started to say "no" because I was afraid of getting more spastic. My brother Dale noticed the way I felt and came into my room. He said, "Gerry, if your God is in fact what you say He is, then He will keep you and give you peace." Suddenly, I knew God would sustain me through this ordeal. He did! So I went into the hospital. On Friday I was wheeled into the operating room. I prayed most earnestly, "Not my will, Lord, but Thy will, be done," and I had peace.

The days following surgery were a hazy blur. I wanted to believe the operation had been successful but sensed this was not so. My left side seemed less capable of responding to my wishes than before. I was disappointed, but I was not angry with God.

Years passed, and gradually my spiritual life came to a standstill. I attended church and read Scripture, but I experienced no joy. I was adrift. I became yet another prodigal son. Oh, I did not waste my substance on riotous living, perhaps because my substance, being a handicapped pension, was rather limited. Nevertheless, I was not living a satisfying life.

I believed in Christ's redemptive power. I knew I had experienced salvation, but I was bothered by the verses in John 10:27,28: *"My sheep listen to my voice; I know them, and they follow me. I give them eternal life, and they shall never perish; no one can snatch them out of my hand."*

I knew I had eternal life and I was secure in His hand, so what then was my problem? I had to ask myself some serious questions. Was I indeed listening to His voice, or was His voice drowned by the other voices I heard all about me? Sheep are to follow their shepherd. How good was I at being a follower of Jesus? Was I following, or was I running ahead? Or worse still, had other paths enticed me?

One Friday night, there was a party going on at the group home. One of the staff attendants, who was also a Christian, reminded me that I also claimed allegiance to Jesus. He bluntly stated, "Remember, Gerry, who your King is. Now suppose you start to show it by your behaviour." I was so angry with him and promptly joined my friends who were drinking in the living room. I did not enjoy the remainder of the evening. What is worse, I did not listen to that person but rather to the other voices I heard about me.

I somehow felt the Lord should strike me down in His anger and take my name out of the Book of Life because of my attitude toward that attendant. But the Lord in His mercy for me, a sinner, sent a young man to work in the group home that fall. He was a new Christian. I couldn't help but notice his Christian life was more joyful than mine. He loved to share Christ with others. I felt I was a "good" Christian because I was attending a Baptist church and had made Jesus my personal Saviour, but what was wrong with me? My new friend asked me to go to his church on a Friday evening. I thought to myself, *I'll go to see his church. I'd like to visit other churches to see how they worship.*

I went to the church via the Disabled Adults Transportation System (DATS) and was met at the door by my friend. He took me into the church basement, and I noticed the people there really loved God in their worship;

they made me feel as if I were in heaven. So I began attending a group of believers in his church on Friday evenings. That young man's love for me made me look at my life according to Christ's standard. I knew my life was not pleasing to my Lord.

As I traveled home from that church on the DATS bus, I felt as if Jesus was sitting across from me. I believe He said, "Take up your cross and stop playing church." I knew I was at a crossroad in my Christian life. Jesus invited me to a closer walk with Him. Right there on that bus, I rededicated my life to God. Shortly afterward, I called my pastor to help me sort out my priorities. I was acutely conscious of God's calling me to change my lifestyle. The following Sunday I publicly rededicated my life to Christ with the prayer, "Take all of my life, Lord; it is yours." I felt peace and joy flood my very being.

Five

Accepting My Relationships

I believe all of us need to have a few good relationships in our life that allow us to be ourselves. We want to have a few people whom we can trust with our lives; they allow us to make mistakes and continue loving us. We also need to have people who can trust us with their life as well.

"The LORD God said, 'It is not good for the man to be alone. I will make a helper suitable for him'" (Genesis 2:18).

The Lord God created woman, for man, so the man would not be lonely. Before this time, the man could talk to God only. But the man needed to have a really good pal or friend to talk with beside God. Such friends might be described as "a touch of God with skin on!"

Some of my friends, both Christians and non-Christians, told me that Christians should not have sexual feelings. Some people even assume that disabled persons do not have such feelings and that we are different in that respect. I need to inform you that, of course, this is not so.

Can you imagine how I felt when my brother dated? I always felt that girls were rather special and fell in and out of love frequently. This often led me to putting my feelings on paper, being misunderstood and then having to recruit my father to go tell my girlfriends when I no longer had special feelings for them.

Why did I have to be buried within my own body? I asked this question of my parents daily. They tried to answer my questions honestly, but I really did not want to hear their answer. I often enjoyed feeling sorry for myself; after all, didn't I have sufficient reason to be despondent? I wallowed in my own despair and self-pity and many times doubted God himself. I became very difficult to live with and often felt spiritually shipwrecked. And yet I realized God does not abandon us.

When my brother Dale got married in Vancouver, I faced, then, what possibly was the hardest time of my life. Our family had driven to Vancouver and stayed with my uncle and aunt prior to the wedding. Their home overlooked the ocean, and we had often enjoyed their hospitality along with the spectacular view.

A few days before the wedding, we had gathered around the dinner table and everyone was talking about the upcoming wedding. I suddenly felt as if someone had plunged a knife into my heart. I was so envious of my brother and his good fortune in finding the girl he wanted to share his life with, that I was completely overcome with jealousy. My anger turned to hate for everyone.

I pushed myself away from the table and hastily went to the TV room. My uncle sensed my feelings and followed me. He tried to talk with me, though he acknowledged he could not possibly understand how I felt. I asked him to leave, because this was something I had to work out with God. I sat looking out at the city lights and had never felt more lonely or desolate in all my life. I began to weep; hot angry tears streamed down my face. When I looked up into the night sky, I heard a voice in my heart, "I know how you feel. God has a plan for you other than marriage."

I had the assurance that His grace was sufficient for even me. Eventually, I rejoined my family and attended the wedding, accepting my new sister-in-law. Now when I look back I am glad that I was not in my brother's shoes because they are now divorced.

A few years later, I met a lady who was in the process of getting a divorce, because her husband was gay. She could not understand him and needed someone to talk to. As a staff member at my group home, she and I became good friends. We could talk about everything, and a few times I shared the gospel with her.

One day I casually asked if she would come out to dinner with me sometime, and she graciously accepted. I made a reservation at a fashionable restaurant.

The setting was lovely, with soft lights, music and good conversation. I felt good inside on that dinner date. She was sitting at a right angle from me, so she could feed me, and I could easily converse with her on my word board. We spoke of many things including Hawaii. What started more as a joke turned into the possibility of a trip to Hawaii together. It ended with her saying she would go with me if I wanted her to. When I looked at her I was surprised to hear myself say, "Yes, come."

Satan had me where I was most vulnerable; my thoughts were on the fun it would be to go to Hawaii with her. I was sure my parents and God would most certainly understand.

However, just before that dinner date, the Missions Committee at my church asked me to type out the opening and

Accepting Life

closing prayers for the service we were planning. I had prepared the opening prayer a few days before. But somehow, no matter how hard I tried over the next few days, I was unable to compose the closing prayer. It crossed my mind to phone the Missions Committee and tell them I could not finish this job! Both the Lord and I knew that my thoughts and motives were not right. So He kept pricking my conscience.

Satan filled my mind with sexual feelings: "Everyone does more than that outside of marriage." Plus, "I gave my word to her that I would be going on that trip with her." I began hoping that my parents would make the decision easier for me, but they simply said they couldn't stop me since I was an adult.

Finally, I shared my dilemma with a friend the following Tuesday evening after Bible study. He heard me out but offered no advice. I felt a little like King David must have felt when the prophet Nathan came to him about Bathsheba. In essence, I had committed adultery with this woman in my heart.

I could have written these words *for myself*:

Have mercy on me, O God, according to your unfailing love; according to your great compassion blot out my transgressions. Wash away all my iniquity and cleanse me from my sin. For I know my transgressions, and my sin is always before me. Against you, you only, have I sinned and done what is evil in your sight, so that you are proved right when you speak and justified when you judge. Surely I was sinful at birth, sinful from the time my mother conceived me (Psalm 51:1–5).

I had to ask myself a lot of questions over that period of the next few days. What if Jesus would return while I was committing this sin? What about the children and the young people in our church, what sort of a witness was I being? I had several very bad days and nights, as my flesh and spirit were at war.

I wanted to get out of this trip, but how? On a Wednesday evening I phoned her, and when I was dialing the phone, I prayed, "Lord, give me a way to get out of this problem." Her husband answered the phone and somehow everything fell into place; I knew my prayer had been answered. I could now back out of the trip arrangement and breathe a prayerful "Thank you." She had wanted to get out of the trip, also, and didn't know how to do that graciously.

The next day I was able to compose that closing prayer I had been struggling with; I believe the Lord washed my sin from me, so I was then able to do so, but, better than that, He even gave me the words for the prayer!

During the Sunday school class, my eyes were filled with tears of joy when I read it. I knew I was loved, and by the very children I had been ready to betray by my sinful actions.

I knew the Lord loved me; I thanked Him that He opened my eyes and directed me. He spared me from doing something I would have eventually regretted. For the first time in many nights I was blessed with a sound and peaceful sleep. Of course I knew all along that to make a trip like that with any girl would be a sin. I realized that once again I had engaged in a real struggle with myself; Satan had been working overtime to break me.

"No temptation has seized you except what is common to man. And God is faithful; he will not let you be tempted beyond what you can bear" (1 Corinthians 10:13).

I still go out on dates, and I enjoy the company of some special ladies. I still hope God will give me someone special who wants to share her life with me. Recently I went to dinner in my friend's home, where she told me she had found Jesus Christ. I was very glad we had not gone to Hawaii together.

Once, I loved a lady that I thought returned my love, and maybe she did. It was possible that because of our love she had not seen my disability. On Christmas Eve we joined my family at my brother's church and then went to my parents for some Christmas goodies. That day, someone's comment made my friend suddenly notice my disability; I heard the statement, "You wouldn't want to be tied down to a disabled man..." I felt the stab of pain, and I knew that my friend was going to think over those words.

It took a while, but on the following Valentine's Day, my lady friend gave me a card at church. However, she asked me not to open the card until I was home. In that card she said goodbye. I wept, because it was so painful; I had deeply loved that woman and her two teenage daughters.

In the hours that followed, I found myself arguing with God. I told Jesus that He just didn't know how painful rejection felt, but in my thoughts He reminded me it had been a friend that turned Him in to the Temple guards with a kiss. He had felt added rejection from most of his friends when He was on trial and again while on the cross for us. Because of carrying our sin, even His Heavenly Father had turned His back on Him, when He was dying on the cross. At this thought, my tears were because of what Jesus had done for me.

Reality still hurt, so I called my parents to come and comfort me, and they did. About one hour later, I heard a child knocking at my door; a friend and his two-year-old son were standing there. Al said that he and his son were taking a ride and noticed they were near my place. He felt that he should stop in and visit with me. His son played with everything he could reach, and that made me laugh again. Once again the Lord showed me His kindness.

Another time I really liked a young lady, but I was afraid she would not go out with me. So an older and wiser man gave me this proverb, "Don't worry if you will have another date with her, but enjoy the moment you have with her." I have forgotten her name, but not the proverb. So now, when I spend time with a friend, I enjoy that moment with him or her, as though I might never again be able to enjoy it again.

From time to time, I have slipped into sin in some of my relationships. Sure, I felt ashamed and disappointed. I can identify with the apostle Paul when he said:

> *"I do not understand what I do. For what I want to do I do not do, but what I hate I do...For I have the desire to do what is good, but I cannot carry it out...Who will rescue me from this body of death? Thanks be to God—through Jesus Christ our Lord!"* (Romans 7:15–25).

A wise old lady was once asked her opinion on whether being single or married was better. She replied, "I would rather wish for what I cannot have, than have what I do not want!" Why is it that we so often want something that we cannot have, rather than being content with what we do have?

I think that when we are not content in our relationships, it is often because we are looking for "greener fields on the other side of the fence." If we seek after those "improvements" they often prove to be a major disappointment. Then, when we want to go back, it is impossible, because everything is different now. We must learn to be satisfied with what we have now. *"I have learned to be content whatever the circumstances"* (Philippians 4:11).

Accepting Life

The first time I saw her was at a party. I knew that Tami was for me; however, she had another boyfriend, who was living here at the group home at that time. I saw something very special in Tami. Sometime later, Tami had an interview to move into this home, and I made sure I was there to interview her. I had made up my mind about Tami then. For the next four or five years our relationship was like a roller coaster ride. I believe there was always a flame of love between us. Sometimes that flame was minimal, but we could not extinguish the flame of love, no matter how we tried. One day I had CMT on while I was at my computer; I saw a video called "I miss my friend." So I went to Tami's room, and I asked her if I could visit with her. Over time our friendship grew into a beautiful relationship, for we fell in love.

One day, I began to miss Tami's company; I wanted to be a friend, nothing more. However, I put a small piece of coal beside the flame; therefore, we started to enjoy each other's company. I began to stay longer each night in her room. Soon we realized that we cared for each other as persons deeply. We had a forest fire of love around us; I enjoy this forest fire.

Tami and I fell in love, and we wanted to get married, Our parents said it was a beautiful idea, but it was impossible for us to do, because of our physical disabilities. We cried together, because we knew this was the truth. We were afraid one of us would walk out of the relationship. Tami knew that she would not walk out, and I knew that I wouldn't walk away from her.

A staff member told me, "Why not be married in your heart to Tami?" I said, "Yes, if she is willing." She went into Tami's room and told her the same thing, and Tami said, "Yes, if he is willing." The staff told Tami that I was willing.

Accepting My Relationships

We decided to buy two rings to remind us and tell the world that we will be faithful and loyal to each other.

That Christmas, Tami went into the Royal Alexendra Hospital; my brother had asked me for Christmas dinner, and Tami told me go to my brother's to have Christmas dinner. My brother changed the time for his dinner, so I could visit with my sweetheart; so I did. I thought, *If this is the last Christmas I have with Tami, then I want to spend Christmas with her.*

The next six months I visited Tami almost daily at the Royal Alexandra Hospital, two care centres and back again to the Royal Alexandra Hospital. Tami's mom and my mom asked me, "Why do you keep going to see Tami daily?" Now I will answer that question; I was afraid of the day when I wouldn't see my sweetheart again until my death. I could not live with my knowing I could have been with Tami more often. Rather, I made the time to visit with Tami whom I loved while she was here. I miss those visits with Tami today. I planted an oak tree in memory of her.

I believe that Tami can now see perfectly, and her hearing is great. Now, Tami is laughing because my grandpa told a story about me. Just maybe, Tami is finding out where London Drugs stores are in heaven, and she will take me along when I get there, because Tami always spent hours in London Drugs at the mall.

Now, I miss my friend Tami, and I will always love her. One day, I will go home to her after my work here is done.

I received two miracles from the Lord. First, the Lord told me to stay with Tami until 9:20 pm; I had booked DATS to pick me up at nine. I stayed with Tami and held her hand; I told her that I loved her. Then I met two ladies, who I now believe were angels, to help me at that late hour get

Accepting Life

on the elevator and phone DATS. Many people are often busy running, but most people are helpful at the elevator or will call DATS for me. The ladies walked slowly at my speed.

The second miracle was when Tami's mom gave me Tami's ashes to be buried. At a care centre, we talked about death. Tami wanted to be buried with me, so I promised her we would. I was unsure Tami's mom would give me Tami's ashes. When I die, my niece Karen will arrange for my burial. How could our desire to be buried together be fulfilled? I thought it was an impossible situation; however, on Friday after Tami's passing away, her mom asked Cindy, the supervisor of the group home, to ask me if I wanted Tami's ashes. Naturally I said yes. I believe the Lord gave Tami's ashes to me so I could keep my promise to Tami.

Six

All Things Work Together for Good

I want to share some thoughts with you on the controversial subject of divine physical healing. I believe that each of us is suffering to some degree or other, whether physically, mentally or emotionally. Most of us at some time or other during a period of crisis have cried out to God, "Why me?" Personally, I struggle with an uncooperative body that does not always respond appropriately to the signals I send it. I have very little motor control, I am unable to use my limbs, I cannot speak and I have to use a word board to communicate; but I can push my wheelchair with my right foot, which gives me a certain amount of independence.

I believe that God could heal me, if that would make me a better vessel for Him. I strove for some time deciding whether or not to put my views in writing. Now that I have, it is my prayer that my readers will draw comfort from these words. I have learned through bittersweet experiences the truth found in the fifth chapter of Paul's letter to the Romans, which tells us that suffering produces endurance, and endurance produces character, and character produces hope, and hope does not disappoint us, because God's love has been poured into our hearts through the Holy Spirit, who has been given to us.

Likewise it was very difficult for me to accept that all things work together for the good of those who love God, to those who are called according to His purpose (Romans 8:28) and to give thanks in everything, for this is the will of God in Christ Jesus concerning you (1 Thessalonians 5:18). However, I do know that God can use me, disabled as I am, for His purpose.

Growing up in my teen years, I felt God did not care for me, and many times I asked of the Lord, and of my mother, the same kind of questions that Job asked.

> *"May the day of my birth perish, and the night it was said 'A boy is born!'...Why were there knees to receive me and breasts that I might be nursed? For now I would be lying down in peace; I would be asleep and at rest with kings and counselors of the earth... Or why was I not hidden in the ground like a stillborn child, like an infant who never saw the light of day? ...Why is light given to those in misery and life to the bitter soul, to those who long for death that does not come, who search for it more than for hidden treasure, who are filled with gladness and rejoice when they reach the grave? Why is life given to a man whose way is hidden, whom God has hedged in? For sighing comes to me instead of food; my groans pour out like water... I have no peace, no quietness; I have no rest, but only turmoil"* (Job 3:3,12–14,16,20-24,26).

I believe some Christians deal with the issue of suffering and healing in a simplistic way. People come up to me and question my faith, because I am in a wheelchair. They keep telling me that if I were a "good" Christian (whatever that means) and had more faith, I would have been physically healed long before now. The question of suffering and healing always goes full circle. Other Christians ask me if I believe that Jesus can heal me. My answer is always that He can heal me, if that is what He wants to do. Invariably they reply that "Yes! Jesus wants to heal you," and then quote, "By His stripes you are healed" (see Isaiah 53:5). But I always ask how they know what God's will is for my life.

Please forgive me if I sound a little weary of these arguments, stated in so many different ways. But I cannot deal with the issue of my disabled body this way; the Lord did not promise that we would have no problems in life, but He did promise sufficient grace for our disabilities. I, through cerebral palsy, have learned to trust God for all my needs, a lesson that perhaps I would have never learned had I been "normal" (whatever that means). I believe the Lord is using me for His glory just the way I am. I believe He is using my disability to help me in my personal spiritual growth, because through it all I am learning to be more understanding and have acquired more patience, kindness and faithfulness.

The apostle Paul had a physical disability and he asked the Lord to remove "the thorn" from his flesh three times, but each time the Lord said, *"My grace is sufficient for you"* (2 Corinthians 12:9). Paul accepted his condition. So, you see, the issue is not one of faith but rather of trust and acceptance. Trusting Him who is almighty and powerful and accepting that which I cannot change is the main issue. In today's society, the image-makers would have us believe we are somehow less acceptable if we are different.

Thank goodness this concept is not God's! As Christians we are, of course, to take special care of our bodies, since they are *"the temple of the Holy Spirit"* (1 Corinthians 6:19). Many is the time I have wished to trade my lot in life with one of my brothers, one who appears whole, but after many struggles and a long walk with God, I have come to accept myself and endeavor to glorify Him in my present state.

So, dear Reader, if you have a disability, please do not let anyone add to your struggles with comfortless words or continuing unhelpful advice. Rather, accept yourself and remind yourself that His grace is sufficient for you.

Seven

Trials & Testings

It is my firm belief that neither sickness, defects nor death were part of God's perfect plan for mankind, for in Genesis we read that God saw all that He had made, and it was good. If this was the case, we must ask ourselves: what went wrong? By the third chapter of Genesis sin had entered, and man had fallen from his first estate with God. That disobedience was subsequently punished. That punishment was a curse, part of which was on his body. From that point on, man's body, created perfect, would now know regression, decay and, finally, death.

The Lord said, *"By the sweat of your brow you will eat your food until you return to the ground, since from it you were taken; for dust you are and to dust you will return"* (Genesis 3:19). And so the Lord God drove the man out of the perfect world and into a world of decay and deterioration as we know it today. Nothing is now perfect; nothing is as God originally wanted it for us.

When, in later times, Jesus came, did He come to redeem our physical bodies? Simply put, the answer is no (not at that point). Jesus came to seek and save that which was lost (Matthew 18:11), and I believe that when Jesus died for us He redeemed us spiritually. If His purpose was to redeem us physically, then Christians should have perfect bodies. Christians should not have sickness, should not have spectacles, hearing aids, walking canes or wheelchairs. They should, in such a case, not see physical death. But these things are not so.

I believe that Jesus will redeem our physical bodies when He comes back to set up His kingdom on earth. The Scriptures say *"And God shall wipe away all tears from their eyes; and there shall be no more death, neither sorrow, nor crying, neither shall there be any more pain: for the former things are passed away"* (Revelation 21:4 KJV).

I have often had sincere Christian encouragement to really pray for a complete physical healing! However, I find that if I keep on praying for such a healing, it shows that I haven't actually accepted reality. The question may be asked whether I am trusting God the way that I should. I would be in essence still arguing with Him, which is sin! The "original manufacturer's instruction manual" says: *"Woe to him who quarrels with his Maker...Does the clay say to the potter what are you making?"* (Isaiah 45:9).

Does this mean a person newly, physically disabled should seek the Lord for healing? I believe the answer is an unqualified Yes! Should parents be seeking God to heal their disabled child? Yes! I believe a person should keep on seeking until God heals or gives the peace and grace to accept what has happened.

James wrote under divine inspiration,

Is anyone among you suffering? Let him pray. Is anyone cheerful? Let him sing psalms. Is anyone among you ill? Let him call for the elders of the church, and let them pray over him anointing him with oil in the name of the Lord. And the prayer of faith will save the sick, and the Lord will raise him up. And if he has committed sin, he will be forgiven (James 5:13–15).

If you feel you have committed a sin that caused your disability, then you should ask the Lord to forgive your sin and He will. He may, or may not, restore your physical body, depending on which will bring the greatest glory to God through your life. Whatever the case, if God chooses not to heal you now, then rejoice for that is the will of God. There are a number of instances in Scripture where we read that God had punished men with illness for their disobedience. Some of the more well known passages are:

Exodus 7–11	The ten plagues
Numbers 12:10–15	Miriam becomes a leper
2 Chronicles 26:16–21	Uzziah's sin, punishment and death
Acts 5:1–10	Ananias & Sapphira lied to the Holy Spirit and died

Just as God punished man's disobedience in those days, so He punishes today with suitable "rods of chastisement"; perhaps the present day epidemic of AIDS would be a good example.

Another example: we have skin cancers, because we are harming our ozone. God placed ozone in the atmosphere to keep the harmful sunrays from us; however, we are destroying it for the sake of a few extra dollars. I believe that we could save our ozone, if we were willing to do that rather than making more money. If we are willing to try to save our ozone, I believe it will be a financial benefit in the long run for our children and our grandchildren.

Did the Lord heal *every* believer in the Scriptures? No! In Paul's second letter to Timothy he mentions that he left Trophimus sick in Miletus. Of course, God may choose to restore the physical body in specific cases for specific reasons. For example, Hezekiah became ill and was at the point of death. He prayed to the Lord, who answered him and gave him a miraculous sign (2 Chronicles 32:24).

Why did Jesus heal some people and not others during His time on earth? The Jews equated sickness with sin; therefore, in order to show He had authority on earth to forgive sin, Jesus would heal the sick. In the Gospel of Mark, the second chapter, we read of the healing of a paralytic man, whose four friends had let down through the roof of the house where Jesus was teaching. When Jesus saw their faith He told the paralytic his sins were forgiven.

> *Immediately Jesus knew in his spirit that this was what they were thinking in their hearts, and he said to them, "Why are you thinking these things? Which is easier: to say to the paralytic, 'Your sins are forgiven,' or to say, 'Get up, take your mat and walk'? But that you may know that the Son of Man has authority on earth to forgive sins ..." He said to the paralytic, "I tell you, get up, take your mat and go home"* (Mark 2:6–11).

Once, I was invited to attend a "coffee house" session at a church where they made much of physical healing. Some of the young people, who were gathered there, told me that if I had more faith in God, then I would be healed. This remark caused much anguish and hurt me deeply. That night, after I returned home, the TV was on in my room and it was tuned to the last part of a Billy Graham program.

I asked the staff to come and turn off the TV, but they

Trials & Testings

were detained. While I was waiting Joni, a quadriplegic, came on as a guest speaker. She said "I do not know why God wanted me in this chair, but He has a special plan for my life."

After the TV was turned off, I cried into my pillow, not for Joni and me, but for those people who make so much of physical healing that they miss the point of why Jesus came to this world. I had given myself over to God long ago, and God spoke through Joni, once again, those words I needed to hear.

Every once in a while I go back to that coffeehouse, and, I am happy to say, now those young people accept me in this chair, just as I am. I believe I am a clay jar and God is the potter. Each of us is different, and God loves each of us. We are just called to a different use.

> *Who are you, O man, to talk back to God? 'Shall what is formed say to him who formed it, "Why did you make me like this?"' Does not the potter have the right to make out of the same lump of clay some for noble purposes and some for common use?* (Romans 9:20–21).

Another time, I was waiting for my ride when a lady, pushing a child in a wheelchair, came up to me and said "Jesus will heal my girl, and Jesus wants to heal you, if only you would believe." Now this sounded nice and the lady meant well, but it made little sense to me, and it is unrealistic to expect to receive a cure for all of the problems in our life.

"*What?*" I thought, "*not again Lord!*" I felt sorry for her because she was looking for an easy answer to the question of why God allowed her child to have cerebral palsy. She invited me to go to her church the following Wednesday, and I accepted her kind invitation.

Afterward, a few people came over to me and said, "If you believe Jesus could heal you, you would be healed." Now, the wisest thing for me to have done at that point was to have said nothing. However, I do love to argue, and so I reproached them for making assumptions regarding my belief, not to mention my relationship with the Lord Jesus Christ.

Pretty soon, the pastor joined in. I noticed he was wearing eyeglasses, so I asked him to explain that if he believed it was a sin for a Christian to have a disability, then why was he wearing glasses? His answer was that he believed he was healed.

"Then why do you wear glasses now?" I asked. He did not have a ready answer, except to say he believed that if we have enough faith we would be healed and that it is between you and God only.

"What about when Peter and John healed a crippled beggar on the steps of the Temple in Acts 3?" I asked. The pastor then tried to explain that the crippled man was asking to be healed when he looked at Peter and John. It is in times like these that we laymen need the gift of discernment, because when looking at that passage of Scripture I cannot see that the crippled man was seeking to be healed.

> *Then Peter said, 'Silver or gold I do not have, but what I have I give you. In the name of Jesus Christ of Nazareth, walk. Taking him by the right hand, he helped him up, and instantly the man's feet and ankles became strong. He jumped to his feet and began to walk. Then he went with them into the temple courts, walking and jumping, and praising God. When all the people saw him walking and praising God, they recognized him as the same man who used to sit begging at the temple gate called Beautiful, and they were filled with wonder and amazement at what had happed to him* (Acts 3:6–10).

The question is whether the disabled beggar looked for God to heal his physical condition? The answer is No! When he saw Peter and John, the disabled man was expecting money from them. Verse 5 states *"so the man gave them his attention, expecting to get something from them."*

Who had the faith to heal that man? Did the beggar, or was it Peter and John who had the faith? I feel the beggar had no faith. It was Peter and John who had the faith; therefore, please do not let anyone tell you that if you had more faith you would be healed. If you ask the Lord to heal you and He doesn't, believe that the Lord wants you just the way you are.

Once again a pastor said, "By His wounds, you have been healed" (Isaiah 53:5). "Sir, you misquoted the Scriptures," I wrote in a letter to him, and the next Sunday, he said, "Thank you for faxing your letter to me. You are right."

Here is that letter that I sent to him:

Pastor,

I am that man who was in a wheelchair. You could hurt disabled persons when you pray for our physical healing. Oh yes, the Lord can heal the physical body, but often the Lord says no because He has different plans for His children. Are you embarrassed when you look at disabled persons or what?

When you said, "By His wounds you have been healed," Sir, you misquoted the Scriptures. It means by His wounds we have been healed from our sins. So, how can you use that verse for our physical healing? I have studied about the doctrine of healing with the best teachers and with God Himself by His Spirit and His Scriptures.

Accepting Life

On Sunday night you forgot to ask me about my spiritual life. I felt you were more interested in my physical health, rather than my spiritual health. May I ask you why? When Jesus was on the earth, He was more interested in a man's spiritual life, rather than His physical body. You might ask me, then, why did Jesus heal so many physical bodies? Jesus wanted to show He could heal our physical bodies, because then we would know Jesus could heal our souls, also; then we could believe in Him and He would give us life, now, and life after death, to whoever believes in Him.

The Lord healed me from death twice, once at birth and once ten years ago. My doctors said it was a miracle ten years ago, because I was at heaven's gate, but my Lord told me it was not yet time for me to depart. That statement hurt me, because I was looking forward to going home, but the Lord told me not yet, because my work on earth was not done. I asked the Lord not to change my physical body, because He would heal me, if I asked, because I am His child. Oh yes, I believe in physical healing through prayer, if it brings glory to God.

So many disabled persons have gotten hurt on that doctrine you have on healing; now I am trying to talk to them and fix their hurting hearts with the Truth of Jesus. Many churches will not like what we say, because it attempts to hit very hard on false doctrines, but Jesus wants us to have true doctrines.

Thank you
Gerry

Trials & Testings

What would Paul think about those Christians who believe that every person who has a physical disability should be seeking for a physical healing? Let us read 1 Corinthians 7:17–24 where Paul wrote:

> *Nevertheless, each one should retain the place in life that the Lord assigned to him and to which God has called him. This is the rule I lay down in all the churches. Was a man already circumcised when he was called? He should not become uncircumcised. Was a man uncircumcised when he was called? He should not be circumcised. Circumcision is nothing, and uncircumcision is nothing. Keeping God's commands is what counts. Each one should remain in the situation which he was in when God called him. Were you a slave when you were called? Don't let it trouble you—although if you can gain your freedom, do so. For he who was a slave when he was called by the Lord is the Lord's freedman; similarly, he who was a free man when he was called is Christ's slave. You were bought at a price; do not become slaves of men. Brothers, each man, as responsible to God, should remain in the situation God called him to.*

Would Paul say to Christians who have a physical disability to be content with their disability? It might bring many more people to Christ. Therefore, rejoice in your physical disability, and again I say, rejoice.

I am always amazed by how stupid some people really seem. They told me, if I were healed I could do more for the Lord, and I would have a better life. I know that the Lord is using me for His glory through my disability, by strengthening other Christians. I am enjoying my life because the

Accepting Life

Lord has blessed me with many good friends; also He seems to provide me with relationships with ladies, who help me to have a more fulfilling life. What more do I need to be happy? I have many children in my life. I am satisfied with my life. May I ask you this question: Are you satisfied with your life?

Did the Lord use a physically disabled person in the Bible? Oh yes, I believe that Moses had some kind of verbal disability. Then why did the Lord not heal Moses rather than having his brother Aaron speak for him? I don't know, and I do not need to know that.

> *Moses said to the* LORD, *"O Lord, I have never been eloquent, neither in the past nor since you have spoken to your servant. I am slow of speech and tongue."*
>
> *The* LORD *said to him, "Who gave man his mouth? Who makes him deaf or mute? Who gives him sight or makes him blind? Is it not I, the* LORD*? Now go; I will help you speak and will teach you what to say."*
>
> *But Moses said, "O Lord, please send someone else to do it."*
>
> *Then the* LORD's *anger burned against Moses and he said, "What about your brother, Aaron the Levite? I know he can speak well. He is already on his way to meet you, and his heart will be glad when he sees you. You shall speak to him and put words in his mouth; I will help both of you speak and will teach you what to do. He will speak to the people for you, and it will be as if he were your mouth and as if you were God to him. But take this staff in your hand so you can perform miraculous signs with it* (Exodus 4:10–17).

Eight

Attitudes

On one occasion my parents were invited as guests at a government-sponsored dinner. Mom was introduced to the various guests, one was the Minister of Health. On being told that her eldest son had a disability, the Minister of Health asked, "Where do you keep him?"

"At home," was the prompt replied. "Oh my, how could you—do you have other children?"

"Yes," my mother said, "I have two other sons".

Shocked, the Minister of Health continued, "Oh my, do you realize what you are doing to them?" He then gave my mother one of *those* looks before mother replied, "Yes I do, and hopefully they will grow-up to be loving, decent, human beings." Those within earshot gasped as she walked away—Mom only smiled.

Another time my friend and I went to a fair on a beautiful July evening to have some fun. Realizing it was time to catch our bus to go home again, I decided to go ahead to catch our ride, while she stopped to buy some candy. That was a dumb mistake, because I took the wrong turn and one

Accepting Life

of my small wheels got jammed in some electric cables on the fair ground.

Someone called St John's Ambulance, and I thought they would help me get out of the cables so I could still catch our ride back home. But I was wrong; these St John's Ambulance volunteers did not understand anything about cerebral palsy. To add to my predicament, I had left my voice box at home. We thought we wouldn't need it, because my friend understood me.

The St John's Ambulance's nurse came with two policemen, and he told the policemen I was having a seizure, so they tied me up—I would think they should know not to tie someone up who is having a seizure. But the policemen were just following orders; I think the police thought the nurse knew what he was doing. They took me into the St John's Ambulance's medical centre on the fairgrounds, just as if I was a "criminal." I felt as if I had been transferred back in time to the Dark Ages, because of the attitudes of the staff and volunteers.

While we were waiting (for one hour) the St John's Ambulance volunteers were discussing openly that the government should really "do away" with all disabled babies when they come into the world. That made me very angry. The female attendant told a sexually explicit joke about some disabled man, right in front of me.

The nurse, finally, got my parents' phone number from me and phoned them to come get me. Dad told him that he was coming; however, my nephew told my father that he would come with them. When Keith came to get me, the nurse told him to go back and get my father. My nephew was not impressed and told the nurse that if he wanted my father then he should go out into the dark and find him. Keith said

Attitudes

that he would stay with me, because he had given his word he would bring Gerry to them. The man finally decided to let Keith take me to my dad.

Before we left, I asked my nephew to call and check on my friend, who had arrived at home; I relaxed a bit after that news and determined that I wanted a few words with "my captor." By having Keith name the letters of the alphabet, I signaled each letter I needed to spell out the phrases. I gave that man a piece of my mind, and I didn't even mind that It took a long time to say it. I'd love to know the version of the story he tells his friends!

When I got back home, I saw my lady friend crying at the back door; she was happy to see me again. Yet, at the same time, she wanted to bawl me out for losing her at the fair ground and making her worry so much about me. When I saw her crying, we exchanged hugs. It was so good to be home again.

Nine

At Heaven's Gate

Attitudes are shaped by our response to experiences. One such significant experience began with a very sharp pain in my left side and my heaving my dinner. The pain felt like somebody had stabbed me with a knife and kept on turning it inside of me. It was absolutely excruciating!

The subsequent frequenting of my doctor's office produced little direction, and I continued to get worse. I felt sleepy much of the time. One night, a staff member asked if I wanted an ambulance. I agreed and asked that my parents be called, but because I presumed I would be returning shortly, I wanted to be dressed properly.

When I got to the hospital, my mom asked me, "How are you?" noting that I was as white as a ghost. I replied that I was fine. But Mom knew that I was very sick. The nursing staff rolled me quickly into an emergency room. They tried putting an oxygen mask on me; however, I kept on removing it. I found it quite frustrating, as I was sure that I didn't need oxygen.

Mom didn't want me to see those "tell-tale" x-rays. However, when she was not looking, I saw good news! I could tell those x-rays were saying I had my "one-way ticket to heaven" virtually in hand!

I know that it was as if I were at the gates of heaven. I wanted to go through those gates. I wanted to go home. But, I heard the loving voice of God saying; "You won't die, not yet." I thought God meant by this I would not die spiritually, but then He explained that I wouldn't experience physical death just then. Oh, I really wanted to argue with the Almighty, because I had seen my x-rays! God probably smiled at me for wanting to disagree with Him.

So, God gave me a vision of the life-support machine that would keep me alive for the next ten days in the ICU. I saw this machine on a white cloud above me in the emergency room. A few days later, when I was in the ICU, my pastor and doctor came to see me, because they thought I only had a few more days. However, I wondered to myself, *"Why are you here? Go visit the sick and dying and let me rest now; we can visit when I am at home again."* I knew that I would live, because God had told me everything would be the same as before. However, my pastor told some of my friends at church that I was dying. The day I was able leave the ICU, I took a look at the life support machine and noticed it was exactly as I had seen it in the vision.

A few days later, Mom sent my youngest brother, Brian, to ask me, "Would you, Gerry, want to be on life support if you ever were to be this ill again?" I spelled out for him, "When I am ninety-eight it will be okay to pull out the plug."

I learned that many people had been praying for me. I asked the Lord why He did not tell the church that I would be okay. He simply reminded me that those people loved me, and they needed to pray for me. Then I understood how prayer works and that the Lord loves to hear His people talk to Him.

I was released on a Friday; I went back home again, telling my doctors that I would stay at home and rest; however, on that Sunday I decided to go to church. It caused a small ruckus because three weeks prior I was supposedly almost dead! Seeing my DATS bus, some people thought it had to be bringing someone else. Some were so sure they were willing to bet on it.

In Acts, we can read a similar story, when Peter was in jail and his friends gathered to pray for him and the Lord answered their prayers. A servant girl went to the door to answer his knock, but when she heard Peter's voice, she was so overjoyed, she forgot to let Peter in. His friends could not believe the servant girl, so "poor" Peter kept on knocking at the door until someone let him in. I would guess that Peter and his friends had many good laughs about it afterward.

My parents were not very surprised when I called them that afternoon and told them I had been at church in the morning. Probably Mom and Dad wondered why I had not gone out somewhere on that Saturday.

Ten

Accepting Reality

Why did God allow me to have cerebral palsy? Please believe me when now I say, "I do not know why." I do not *want* to know why I have cerebral palsy; I do not need to know that answer: all I need is to trust Him, to believe I am glorifying God through my life. People often ask me, how I thank God for my cerebral palsy body. Well cerebral palsy does not glorify God, but I am not the cerebral palsy; I have cerebral palsy the same way some people have poor eyesight and need glasses.

I feel my affliction helps me to be a better Christian. Sometimes it helps other Christians to be more like Christ and that, my friends, is how I can glorify God with my cerebral palsy body.

I believe that when God our Father looks down on me, I am perfect in His sight; I have a perfect mind, spirit and body because I am in Christ. Paul wrote, *"If anyone is in Christ, he is a new creation; the old has gone, the new has come!"* (2 Corinthians 5:17). I have cerebral palsy now, but I have the hope I will some day have a new body.

Accepting Life

Peter wrote these words: *"he himself bore our sins in his body on the tree, so that we might die to sins and live for righteousness; by his wounds you have been healed"* (1 Peter 2:24). There are those who think those verses apply to this present time on earth and, if God seemingly does not heal them, then they believe they have insufficient faith to be healed. This is not so; it is simply their misinterpretation of the Scriptures.

I believe these verses look toward the time of the new beginning, when the Lord will bring the new heaven and the new earth; it is written there will be no more death or suffering or disability, for those things have passed away (Revelation 21:4). In the meantime, however, we must learn to live with our imperfect bodies and trust God to give us His sufficient grace.

I am asking you to accept me, just as I am. I have learned to accept that which God has given me. Can you accept that which God has given to us? God gave us His Son that we might have life and have it more abundantly. If you are not a Christian and you want to have what I have and share in that abundant life, why not ask Jesus to come into your life. May I help you to pray to be 100 percent spiritually healed?

Please pray this prayer with me: "Jesus, I am a sinner. Please deliver me from the bondage of Satan. I know that I am going on the wrong path and I ask you, Jesus, to forgive me of my sins, and please, Lord, help me to live with my disability. Thank you, Lord. Amen."

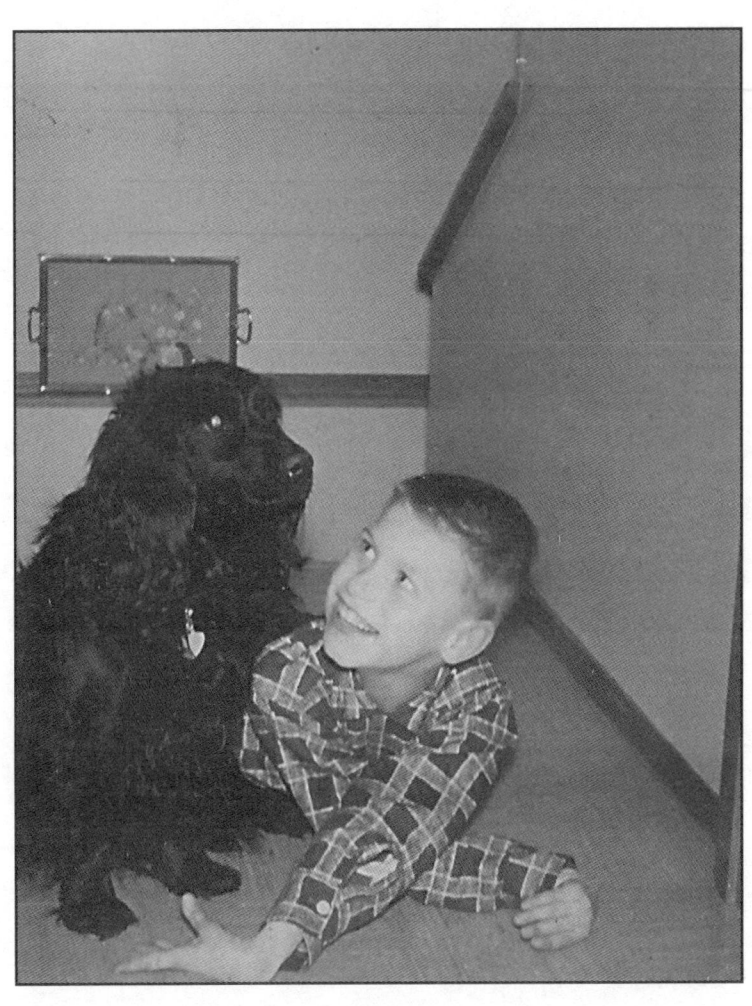

Gerry and Jet

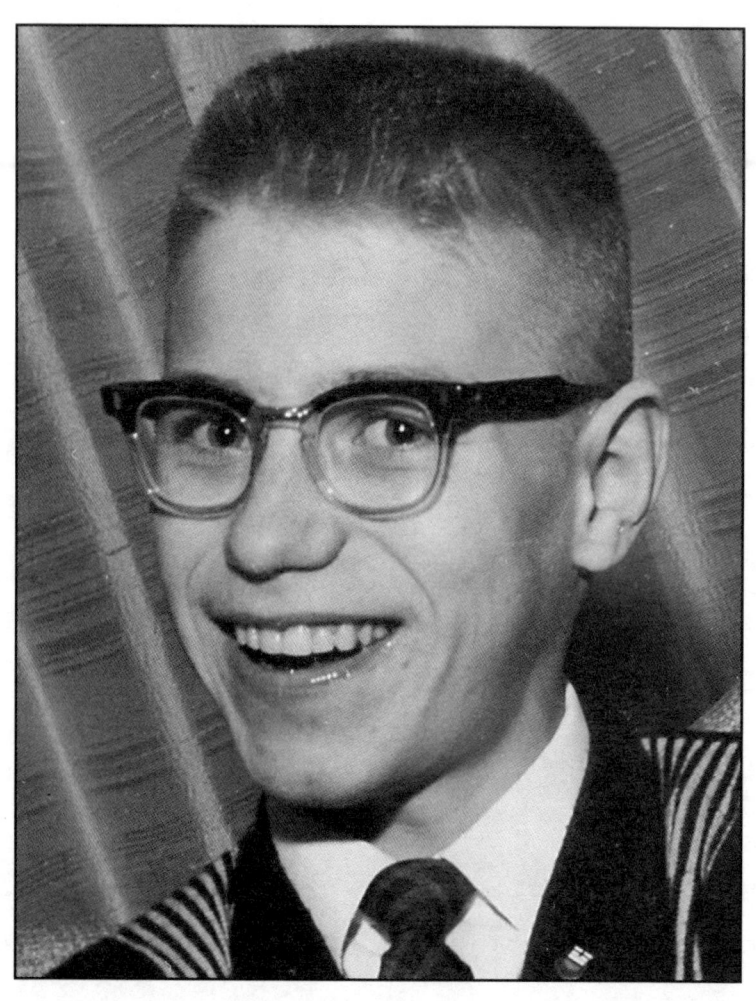

Gerry, age fifteen

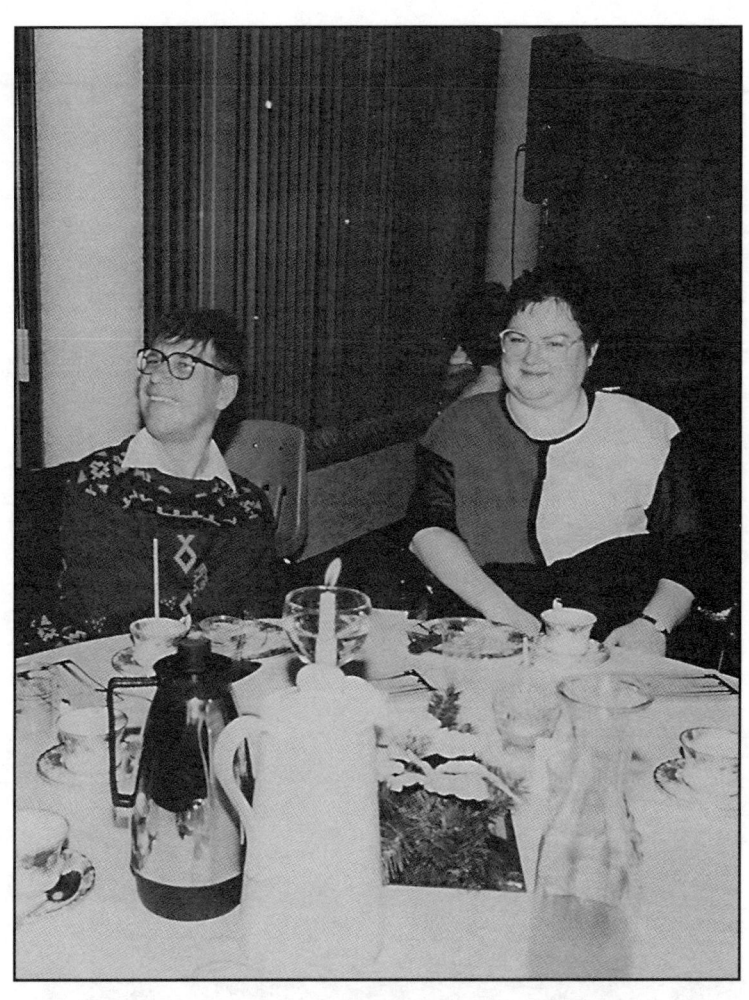

Gerry and Tami

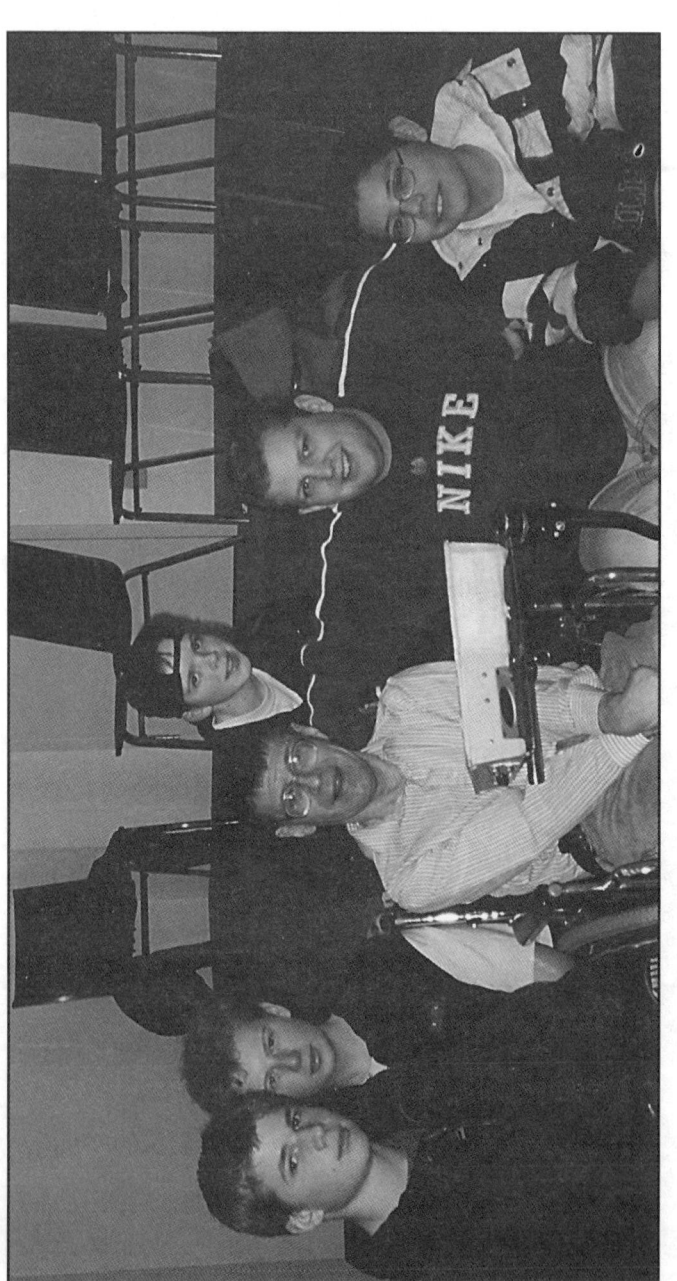

Gerry and his boys' group